Positive affirmations

CW00401372

Trying to conceive can be a stressful and heartbreaking time for many couples, and while it's easy to get disheartened, keeping a positive mindset can actually have a huge impact on the odds of conception.

Of course, positivity isn't the answer to all fertility problems, but it can really help couples to keep focused and optimistic through whatever challenge they face, reframe their experiences and express gratitude for all that they have - and are hoping for.

While self-care and journaling can be a good place to start, so too can positive affirmations. In this book you'll find 30 positive mantras for fertility along with further blank pages for you to add some more of your own, create a vision board or keep a gratitude journal.

You'll also find the details of charities and support networks who can help you on your fertility journey.

We hope you find these a valuable tool, and send lots of positive vibes your way.

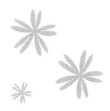

The little book of

Fertility Affirmations

to boost positivity and support mental health
when trying to conceive

Keeping Mum Press, 2022

I am
grateful
for my
body

I have everything I need to grow a healthy baby

I am happy.
I am
healthy.
I am ready.

My body
has the
power to
heal

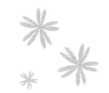

I am
thankful
for the time
to prepare
my body

My body
was
made
for this

I am grateful for the opportunity to become a parent

I am patient with those around me who don't understand my struggle

Today
I am
filled
with
hope

I am
not
alone
in this
process

Love
surrounds me
and the
universe
supports me
in getting
pregnant

Motherhood
is my
destiny

It's okay for pregnancy to take a while

I will
conceive a
healthy,
happy baby

I can't wait
to experience
the miracle
of pregnancy
and
childbirth

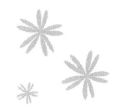

I nourish myself with healthy things that will help me to conceive

My partner
and I are
supportive
of each other
in this
journey

Pregnancy is possible for me

My body
is in
tune with
what it needs
to become
pregnant

I am
made
for
motherhood

Whatever
the
outcome,
I will
survive

I cannot control everything, and that is okay

I am
surrounded
by those
who love,
support and
respect me

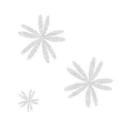

I am
making
the best
choices for
my body

I put my faith and trust into the power within my body

I celebrate
every
cycle
as a new
opportunity

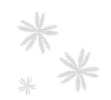

I am
strong
and
capable

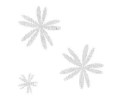

Patience and care help prepare my body for pregnancy

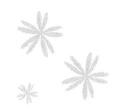

I will
conceive
at the
perfect
time

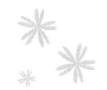

I know
my body
is
working
perfectly

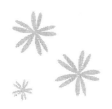

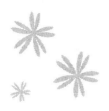

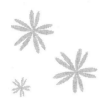

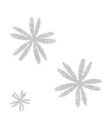

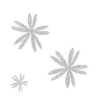

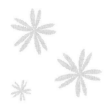

Resources for Fertility Advice and Support

Fertility Network
fertilitynetworkuk.org

The Fertility Foundation UK
fertilityfoundation.org

Resolve
resolve.org

Printed in Great Britain
by Amazon

21918755R00042